Diabetic Renal Diet Cookbook

Hector A. Anderson

Table of Contents

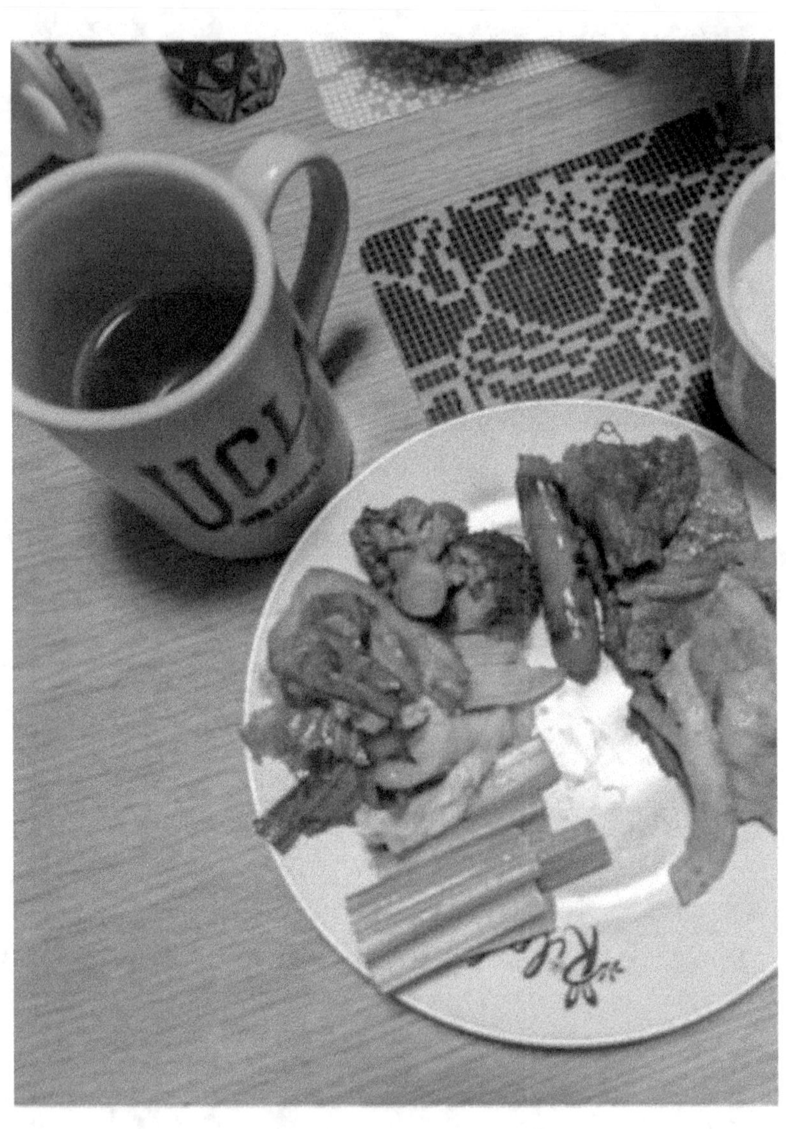

Introduction

This book has been carefully crafted to provide you with a collection of delicious and nutritious recipes tailored specifically for individuals with diabetes and renal (kidney) conditions. We understand the challenges you may face in managing your dietary needs, and our goal is to help you navigate your health journey while still enjoying satisfying and flavorful meals.

Living with diabetes and renal issues requires a thoughtful approach to nutrition. It is essential to strike a balance between managing blood sugar levels and supporting optimal kidney function. The recipes within this cookbook have been thoughtfully designed to address these dual needs, offering a wide range of flavorful dishes that are not only kidney-friendly but also suitable for individuals with diabetes.

In this book you will find a diverse selection of recipes for breakfast, lunch, and dinner, as well as snacks and desserts. Each recipe is accompanied by a list of ingredients and clear step-by-step instructions to ensure ease of preparation. We have carefully chosen ingredients that are low in sodium, rich in essential nutrients, and suitable for individuals with renal and diabetic dietary restrictions.

In addition to providing nourishing recipes, this book aims to empower you with valuable information about the benefits of a diabetic renal diet. You will discover how certain food choices can positively impact your blood sugar levels and support kidney health. We have also included tips on meal planning, portion control, and smart substitutions to help you make informed decisions about your diet.

We understand that embarking on a new dietary regimen can be challenging, but we want to assure you that you are not alone on this journey. Alongside the recipes, you will find practical advice, guidance, and encouragement to help you stay motivated and focused on your health goals.

It is our sincere hope this cookbook becomes your go-to resource for delicious, kidney-friendly meals that support your diabetic management. With the right tools, knowledge, and flavorful recipes at your disposal, you can embark on a culinary adventure that will nourish your body, please your taste buds, and contribute to your overall well-being.

Remember, nourishing your body is an act of self-care, and by embracing this cookbook, you are taking a significant step towards a healthier and happier life. Let's embark on this culinary journey together and make every meal a nourishing and enjoyable experience.

Chapter 1

About Diabetic Renal Disease

Diabetic renal disease, also known as diabetic nephropathy, is a common complication of diabetes mellitus that affects the kidneys. It is a leading cause of chronic kidney disease (CKD) and end-stage renal disease (ESRD) worldwide.

Diabetes mellitus is a chronic metabolic disorder characterized by high blood sugar levels due to insufficient insulin production or impaired insulin function. Over time, uncontrolled diabetes can damage various organs, including the kidneys.

Diabetic renal disease typically develops after several years of having diabetes, especially if blood sugar levels are poorly controlled. The exact cause of this condition is not fully understood, but it is believed to be multifactorial. Elevated blood sugar levels can lead to the accumulation of glucose in the kidneys, causing damage to the blood vessels and filtration units of the kidneys called nephrons.

The progression of diabetic renal disease can be divided into several stages. Initially, there may be an increase in the filtration rate of the kidneys, leading to the leakage of small amounts of protein, known as microalbuminuria. As the disease progresses, larger amounts of protein, called macroalbuminuria, may be excreted in the urine. Eventually, the kidneys' ability to filter waste products and excess fluid decreases, leading to a condition known as end-stage renal disease.

Symptoms of diabetic renal disease may include swelling in the legs, ankles, feet, or face, increased blood pressure, foamy or frothy urine, fatigue, nausea, and a decreased appetite. However, there may be no visible signs in the early stages.

Prevention and management of diabetic renal disease primarily involve controlling blood sugar levels and managing other risk factors such as hypertension and dyslipidemia. Treatment may include lifestyle modifications such as a healthy diet, regular exercise, weight management, and smoking cessation. Medications such as angiotensin-converting enzyme (ACE) inhibitors or angiotensin receptor blockers (ARBs) are commonly prescribed to control blood pressure and reduce proteinuria.

In advanced stages of diabetic renal disease, dialysis or kidney transplantation may be necessary to sustain life. Therefore, early detection and appropriate management of diabetes are crucial to prevent or delay the onset of diabetic renal disease and its complications. Regular monitoring of kidney function through urine tests and blood tests is recommended for individuals with diabetes. Consultation with a healthcare professional, such as a primary care physician or endocrinologist, is essential for the diagnosis, treatment, and ongoing management of diabetic renal disease.

Chapter 2

How to Follow Diabetic Renal Diets

To follow a diabetic renal diet, here are some general guidelines:

1. **Work with a healthcare professional:** Consult a registered dietitian or healthcare provider who specializes in diabetic renal diets. They will assess your specific needs, provide personalized guidance, and help create a meal plan that suits your condition, taking into account your kidney function, blood sugar levels, and other health factors.

2. **Control carbohydrate intake:** Monitor and distribute your carbohydrate intake throughout the day to manage blood sugar levels. Choose complex carbohydrates like whole grains, legumes, and vegetables over processed carbohydrates since they have a slower effect on blood sugar. Avoid sugary foods and beverages that can cause rapid spikes in blood sugar.

3. **Limit sodium intake:** Reduce your consumption of processed and packaged foods, as they tend to be high in sodium. Opt for fresh, unprocessed foods, and use herbs, spices, and other seasonings to add flavor to your meals instead of relying on salt. This aids in the regulation of blood pressure and fluid retention.

4. Moderate protein intake: Depending on your kidney function, your healthcare provider may recommend a controlled protein intake. They will determine the appropriate amount of protein to limit stress on the kidneys while ensuring you still meet your nutritional needs. Focus on high-quality protein sources such as lean meats, fish, poultry, eggs, and plant-based proteins like legumes and tofu.

5. Monitor fluid intake: If you have fluid restrictions, follow the recommended daily fluid limit provided by your healthcare provider. Be mindful of your fluid intake from beverages and foods, including soups, fruits, and vegetables with high water content. Measure and keep track of your fluid intake to stay within the recommended limits.

6. Balance macronutrients: Aim for a well-balanced diet that includes a combination of carbohydrates, proteins, and healthy fats. This helps provide essential nutrients while supporting blood sugar control and overall health.

7. Pay attention to portion sizes: Be mindful of portion sizes to manage calorie intake and maintain a healthy weight. Use measuring cups, a food scale, or other portion control tools to ensure you're consuming appropriate amounts of food.

Benefits of following a diabetic renal diet:

1. Blood sugar control: The diet helps regulate blood sugar levels, reducing the risk of further kidney damage and other complications associated with uncontrolled diabetes.

2. Blood pressure management: By reducing sodium intake and promoting a balanced diet, the diet helps control blood pressure, preventing additional strain on the kidneys.

3. Kidney function preservation: Following a diabetic renal diet can slow the progression of kidney damage and preserve kidney function, improving long-term outcomes.

4. Nutritional support: The diet focuses on providing essential nutrients while considering the specific needs of individuals with diabetic renal disease. It helps prevent nutrient deficiencies and supports overall health.

5. Weight management: The diet emphasizes portion control and healthy food choices, promoting weight management. Maintaining a healthy weight can improve insulin sensitivity, blood sugar control, and overall kidney function.

6. Reduced fluid retention: By monitoring fluid intake, the diet helps manage fluid retention, reducing swelling, high blood pressure, and discomfort.

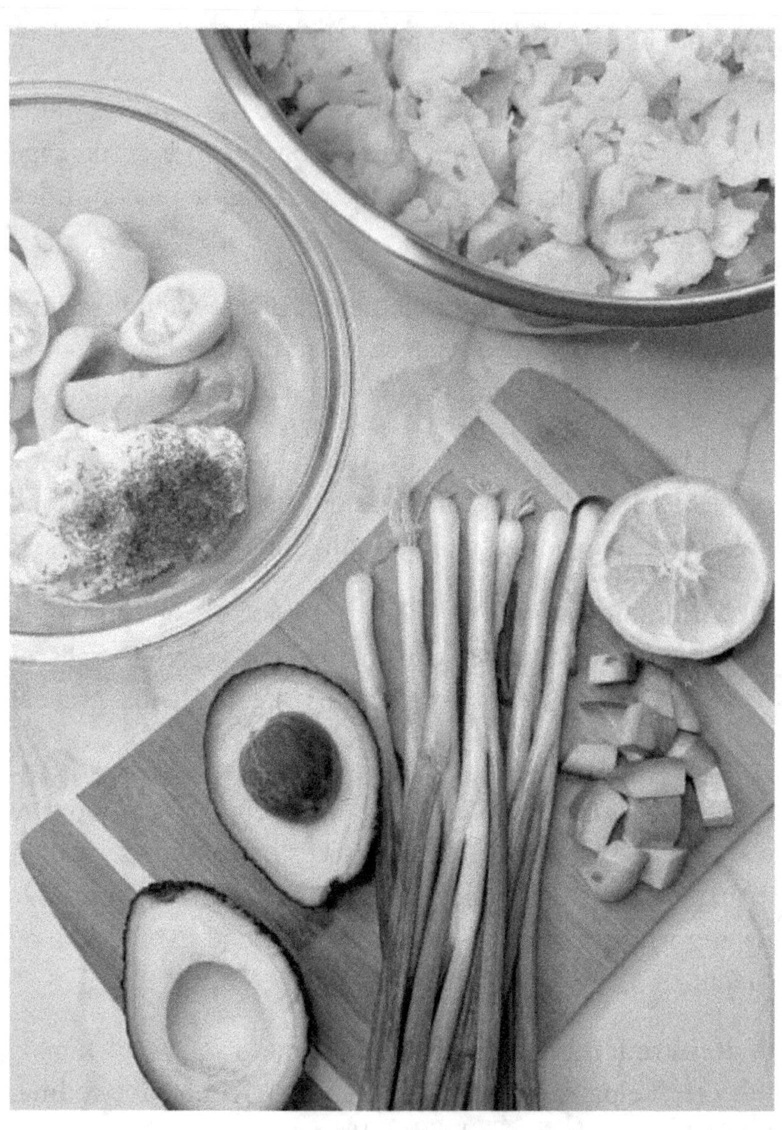

Chapter3

7 Days Meal Plan for Diabetic Renal Diet

Here's a 7-day meal plan for a diabetic renal diet:

Day 1:

Breakfast:

- Egg white scrambled with spinach and tomatoes
- Whole grain toast
- Sliced peaches

Lunch:

- Grilled chicken breast
- Quinoa salad with cucumber, cherry tomatoes, and lemon vinaigrette
- Steamed green beans

Snack:

- Carrot sticks with hummus

Dinner:

- Baked salmon with herbs and lemon
- Brown rice

- Steamed asparagus

Day 2:

Breakfast:

- Oatmeal with mixed berries and chopped almonds

- Unsweetened almond milk

Lunch:

- Avocado and turkey wrapped up with whole wheat tortilla

- Mixed green salad with balsamic vinaigrette

Snack:

- Greek yogurt with sliced almonds

Dinner:

- Grilled shrimp skewers

- Quinoa pilaf with mixed vegetables

- Steamed broccoli

Day 3:

Breakfast:

- Veggie and cheese omelette with bell peppers, onions, and mushrooms

- Whole grain toast

- Orange slices

Lunch:

- Lentil soup

- Spinach salad with cherry tomatoes and lemon-tahini dressing

Snack:

- Apple slices with almond butter

Dinner:

- Baked chicken breast

- Barley salad with roasted vegetables

- Steamed Brussels sprouts

Day 4:

Breakfast:

- Greek yogurt with fresh berries and a sprinkle of flaxseeds

- Whole grain crackers

Lunch:

- Grilled tofu with teriyaki sauce

- Brown rice

- Stir-fried mixed vegetables

Snack:

- Celery sticks with peanut butter

Dinner:

- Baked cod with herbs and lemon

- Quinoa with sautéed mushrooms and onions

- Steamed cauliflower

Day 5:

Breakfast:

- Vegetable and feta cheese frittata

- Whole grain English muffin

- Grapefruit segments

Lunch:

- Turkey chili with kidney beans and diced tomatoes

- Mixed green salad with vinaigrette dressing

Snack:

- Cottage cheese with pineapple chunks

Dinner:

- Baked pork tenderloin with rosemary

- Barley pilaf with sautéed zucchini and bell peppers

- Steamed green beans

Day 6:

Breakfast:

- Egg whites scrambled with spinach and tomatoes

- Whole grain toast

- Sliced strawberries

Lunch:

- Grilled chicken breast

- Quinoa salad with cucumber, cherry tomatoes, and lemon vinaigrette

- Steamed asparagus

Snack:

- Carrot sticks with hummus

Dinner:

- Baked salmon with herbs and lemon

- Brown rice

- Roasted Brussels sprouts

Day 7:

Breakfast:

- Oatmeal with mixed berries and chopped almonds

- Unsweetened almond milk

Lunch:

- Avocado and turkey wrapped with whole wheat tortilla

- Mixed green salad with balsamic vinaigrette

Snack:

- Greek yogurt with sliced almonds

Dinner:

- Grilled shrimp skewers

- Quinoa pilaf with mixed vegetables

- Steamed broccoli

Remember to adjust portion sizes and specific ingredients according to your dietary needs and any recommendations from your healthcare provider.

Chapter 4

10 Diabetic Renal Breakfast Recipes

Here are ten diabetic renal breakfast recipes along with their ingredients and preparation methods:

1. Spinach and Mushroom Egg White Omelette:

Ingredients:

- 4 egg whites

- Handful of fresh spinach

- Sliced mushrooms

- Salt and pepper to taste

- Cooking spray

Preparation:

1. In a bowl, whisk the egg whites until frothy.

2. Heat a non-stick pan over medium heat and lightly coat with cooking spray.

3. Add the sliced mushrooms to the pan and sauté for a few minutes until tender.

4. Cook the spinach until it is wilted in the pan.

5. Pour the whisked egg whites over the vegetables in the pan.

6. Cook until the omelette is set and lightly golden on both sides.

7. Add salt and pepper to taste and serve.

2. Berry and Almond Overnight Oats: Ingredients:

- ½ cup rolled oats

- ½ cup unsweetened almond milk

- ½ cup mixed berries (strawberries, blueberries, raspberries)

- 1 tablespoon chopped almonds

- 1 teaspoon chia seeds (optional)

- ½ teaspoon honey or sweetener of choice (optional)

Preparation:

1. In a jar or bowl, combine the rolled oats and almond milk.

2. Stir in the mixed berries, chopped almonds, chia seeds (if using), and sweetener (if desired).

3. Cover and refrigerate overnight.

4. In the morning, give the mixture a stir and enjoy chilled.

3. Greek Yogurt Parfait:

Ingredients:

- ½ cup plain Greek yogurt

- ¼ cup mixed berries (strawberries, blueberries, raspberries)

- 1 tablespoon chopped walnuts

- Optional: 1 teaspoon of honey or sweetener of choice

Preparation:

1. In a glass or bowl, layer the Greek yogurt, mixed berries, and chopped walnuts.

2. Drizzle honey or add a sweetener of choice (if desired).

3. Repeat the layers.

4. Serve immediately.

4. Veggie Breakfast Wrap:

Ingredients:

- 1 whole wheat tortilla

- 2 egg whites, scrambled

- Handful of baby spinach

- Sliced bell peppers

- Sliced tomatoes

- Salt and pepper to taste

Preparation:

1. Heat the tortilla in a dry pan or microwave until pliable.

2. Layer the scrambled egg whites, baby spinach, sliced bell peppers, and sliced tomatoes on the tortilla.

3. Season with salt and pepper.

4. Roll the tortilla tightly into a wrap.

5. Slice in half and enjoy.

5. Quinoa Breakfast Bowl:

Ingredients:

- ½ cup cooked quinoa

- ¼ cup unsweetened almond milk

- 1 tablespoon chopped almonds

- 1 tablespoon dried cranberries

- Optional: 1 teaspoon of honey or sweetener of choice

Preparation:

1. In a bowl, combine the cooked quinoa and almond milk.

2. Stir in the chopped almonds, dried cranberries, and sweetener (if desired).

3. Microwave for 1-2 minutes until warm.

4. Give it a stir and enjoy.

6. Avocado and Tomato Toast:

Ingredients:

- 1 slice whole grain bread, toasted

- ¼ ripe avocado, mashed

- Sliced tomatoes

- Salt and pepper to taste

Preparation:

1. Spread the mashed avocado on the toasted bread.

2. Top with sliced tomatoes.

3. Season with salt and pepper.

4. Serve and enjoy.

7. Cottage Cheese and Fruit Bowl:

Ingredients:

- ½ cup low-fat cottage cheese

- Assorted fresh fruits (such as berries, sliced kiwi, and grapes)

- Chopped nuts 1 tablespoon (Like almonds or walnuts)

- Cinnamon (optional)

Preparation:

1. Place the cottage cheese in a mixing basin.

2. Top with fresh fruits and chopped nuts.

3. Sprinkle with cinnamon (if desired).

4. Serve chilled.

8. Vegetable Frittata Muffins:

Ingredients:

- 4 eggs

- Vegetables (such as bell peppers, onions, and spinach) chopped

- Salt and pepper to taste

- Cooking spray

Preparation:

1. Preheat the oven to 350°F (175°C) and grease a muffin tin with cooking spray.

2. In a bowl, whisk the eggs until well-beaten.

3. Stir in the chopped vegetables, salt, and pepper.

4. Pour the egg mixture evenly into the greased muffin tin.

4. Bake for approximately 15-20 minutes or until the frittata muffins are set and lightly golden.

5. Allow them to cool slightly before removing from the muffin tin.

6. Serve warm or refrigerate and enjoy throughout the week.

9. Chia Pudding:

Ingredients:

- 2 tablespoons chia seeds

- ½ cup unsweetened almond milk

- ¼ teaspoon vanilla extract

- Optional; 1 teaspoon honey or sweetener of choice.

- Sliced fruits for topping (such as berries or bananas)

Preparation:

1. In a jar or bowl, combine the chia seeds, almond milk, vanilla extract, and sweetener (if desired).

2. Stir well to ensure the chia seeds are evenly distributed.

3. Cover and refrigerate for at least 2 hours or overnight, stirring occasionally..

4. When ready to serve, top with sliced fruits.

10. Smoothie Bowl:

Ingredients:

- 1 ripe banana

- ½ cup mixed berries (such as strawberries, blueberries, and raspberries)

- ½ cup unsweetened almond milk

- 1 tablespoon nut butter (such as almond or peanut butter)

- Toppings of choice (such as chopped nuts, seeds, or shredded coconut)

Preparation:

1. In a blender, combine the banana, mixed berries, almond milk, and nut butter.

2. Blend until smooth and creamy.

3. Pour the smoothie into a bowl.

4. Top with your favorite toppings.

5. Enjoy with a spoon.

Remember to adjust the portion sizes and specific ingredients according to your dietary needs and any recommendations from your healthcare provider. Enjoy these breakfast recipes as part of a balanced diabetic renal diet.

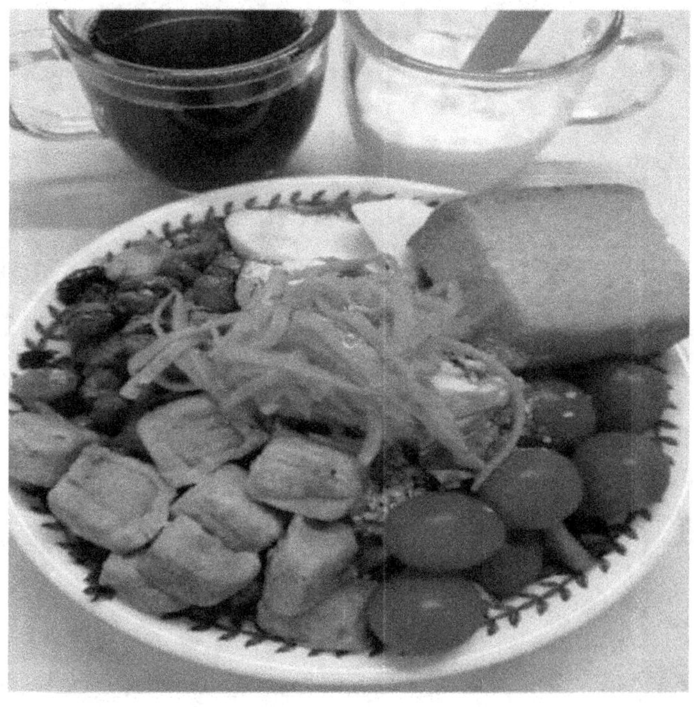

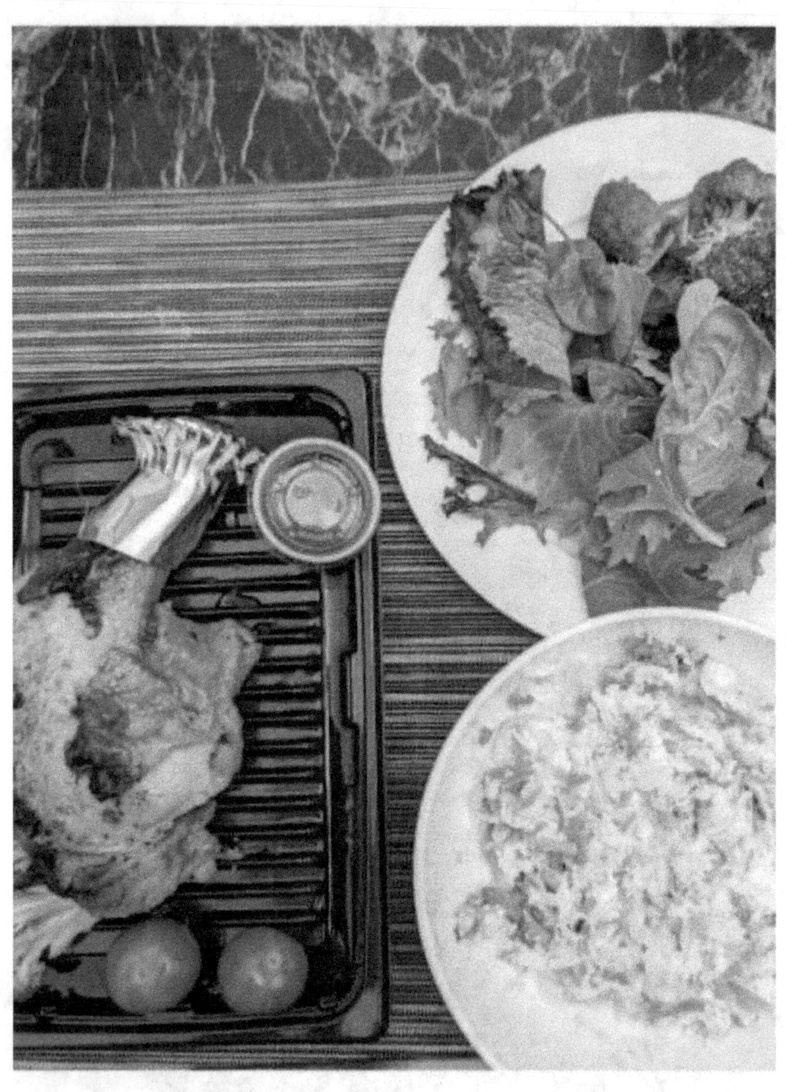

Chapter 5

10 Diabetic Renal Lunch Recipes

Here are ten diabetic renal lunch recipes along with their ingredients and preparation methods:

1. Grilled Chicken Salad:

Ingredients:

- Grilled chicken breast, sliced

- Mixed salad greens

- Cucumber, sliced

- Cherry tomatoes, halved

- Red onion, thinly sliced

- Olive oil and vinegar dressing (low-sodium)

- Salt and pepper to taste

Preparation:

1. In a large bowl, combine the mixed salad greens, cucumber slices, cherry tomatoes, and red onion.

2. Top with sliced grilled chicken breast.

3. Drizzle with olive oil and vinegar dressing.

4. Season with salt and pepper.

5. Toss to coat all the ingredients.

6. Serve chilled.

2. Quinoa and Vegetable Stir-Fry:

Ingredients:

- Cooked quinoa

- Assorted vegetables (such as bell peppers, broccoli, and snap peas)

- Low-sodium soy sauce

- Garlic powder

- Ginger powder

- Olive oil

Preparation:

1. Heat olive oil in a skillet or wok over medium-high heat.

2. Add the assorted vegetables to the skillet and stir-fry until tender-crisp.

3. Stir in the cooked quinoa.

4. Season with garlic powder and ginger powder.

5. Stir in low-sodium soy sauce.

6. Cook for a few more minutes until the flavors are well combined.

7. Serve hot.

3. Tuna Salad Lettuce Wraps:

Ingredients:

- Canned tuna in water, drained
- Greek yogurt (plain, non-fat)
- Diced celery
- Diced red bell pepper
- Diced red onion
- Lemon juice
- Salt and pepper to taste
- Lettuce leaves

Preparation:

1. In a bowl, combine the canned tuna, Greek yogurt, diced celery, diced red bell pepper, diced red onion, lemon juice, salt, and pepper.

2. Mix until all of the ingredients are uniformly distributed.

3. Spoon the tuna salad onto lettuce leaves.

4. Roll the lettuce leaves to form wraps.

5. Serve chilled.

4. Lentil and Vegetable Soup:

Ingredients:

- Green or brown lentils, rinsed

- Assorted vegetables (such as carrots, celery, and zucchini), diced

- Onion, chopped

- Garlic cloves, minced

- Low-sodium vegetable broth

- Dried thyme

- Olive oil

- Salt and pepper to taste

Preparation:

1. In a large pot, heat the olive oil over medium heat..

2. Sauté the chopped onion, minced garlic, and diced vegetables until softened.

3. Add the rinsed lentils, low-sodium vegetable broth, dried thyme, salt, and pepper.

4. Bring to a boil, then reduce the heat and simmer for 25-30 minutes or until the lentils are tender.

5. Adjust seasoning if needed.

6. Serve hot.

5. Grilled Vegetable Wrap:

Ingredients:

- Assorted vegetables (such as bell peppers, zucchini, and eggplant), sliced

- Whole wheat tortilla

- Hummus (low-sodium)

- Fresh spinach leaves

- Salt and pepper to taste

Preparation:

1. Preheat the grill or grill pan on medium-high heat.

2. Grill the sliced vegetables until tender and lightly charred.

3. Spread a layer of hummus on a whole wheat tortilla.

4. Layer fresh spinach leaves and grilled vegetables on top.

5. Season with salt and pepper.

6. Roll the tortilla tightly into a wrap.

7. Slice in half and serve.

6. Shrimp and Vegetable Stir-Fry:

Ingredients:

- Shrimp, peeled and deveined

- Assorted vegetables (such as bell peppers, broccoli, and snap peas)

- Low-sodium soy sauce

- Garlic powder

- Ginger powder

- Olive oil

Preparation:

1. Heat olive oil in a skillet or wok over medium-high heat.

2. Add the shrimp to the skillet and cook until pink and opaque.

3. Remove the cooked shrimp from the skillet and set aside.

4. In the same skillet, add the assorted vegetables and stir-fry until tender-crisp.

5. Put the cooked shrimp back in the skillet.

6. Season with garlic powder and ginger powder.

7. Stir in low-sodium soy sauce.

8. Cook for a few more minutes until the flavors are well combined.

9. Serve hot over brown rice or quinoa.

7. Chicken and Vegetable Stir-Fry:

Ingredients:

- Skinless, boneless chicken breast, sliced

- Assorted vegetables (such as bell peppers, broccoli, and carrots), sliced

- Low-sodium soy sauce

- Garlic powder

- Ginger powder

- Olive oil

Preparation:

1. Heat olive oil in a skillet or wok over medium-high heat.

2. Add the sliced chicken breast to the skillet and cook until browned and cooked through.

3. Set aside the cooked chicken from the skillet.

4. In the same skillet, add the assorted vegetables and stir-fry until tender-crisp.

5. Put the cooked chicken back in the skillet.

6. Season with garlic powder and ginger powder.

7. Stir in low-sodium soy sauce.

8. Cook for a few more minutes until the flavors are well combined.

9. Serve hot over brown rice or quinoa.

8. Spinach and Mushroom Omelette:

Ingredients:

- Eggs

- Fresh spinach leaves

- Sliced mushrooms

- Onion, chopped

- Salt and pepper to taste

- Cooking spray

Preparation:

1. Heat a non-stick skillet over medium heat and coat with cooking spray.

2. Sauté the chopped onion and sliced mushrooms until softened.

3. Add the fresh spinach leaves to the skillet and cook until wilted.

4. In a separate bowl, beat the eggs with salt and pepper.

5. Pour the beaten eggs over the cooked vegetables in the skillet.

6. Cook until the omelette is set and lightly golden on the bottom.

7. Flip the omelette and cook for a few more minutes.

8. Fold the omelette in half and serve hot.

9. Greek Salad with Grilled Chicken:

Ingredients:

- Grilled chicken breast, sliced

- Mixed salad greens

- Cucumber, sliced

- Cherry tomatoes, halved

- Kalamata olives, pitted

- Red onion, thinly sliced

- Feta cheese, crumbled

- Olive oil and lemon dressing (low-sodium)

- Salt and pepper to taste

Preparation:

1. In a large bowl, combine the mixed salad greens, cucumber slices, cherry tomatoes, Kalamata olives, red onion, and crumbled feta cheese.

2. Top with sliced grilled chicken breast.

3. Drizzle with olive oil and lemon dressing.

4. Season with salt and pepper.

5. Toss to coat all the ingredients.

6. Serve chilled.

10. Mexican Black Bean and Corn Salad:

Ingredients:

- Black beans, cooked and rinsed

- Corn kernels (fresh or frozen)

- Red bell pepper, diced

- Red onion, diced

- Cilantro leaves, chopped

- Lime juice

- Olive oil

- Cumin powder

- Salt and pepper to taste

Preparation:

1. In a bowl, combine the black beans, corn kernels, diced red bell pepper, diced red onion, and chopped cilantro leaves.

2. Drizzle with lime juice and olive oil.

3. Sprinkle cumin powder, salt, and pepper.

4. Toss to coat all the ingredients.

5. Serve chilled.

Remember to adjust the portion sizes and specific ingredients according to your dietary needs and any recommendations from your healthcare provider. Enjoy these lunch recipes as part of a balanced diabetic renal diet.

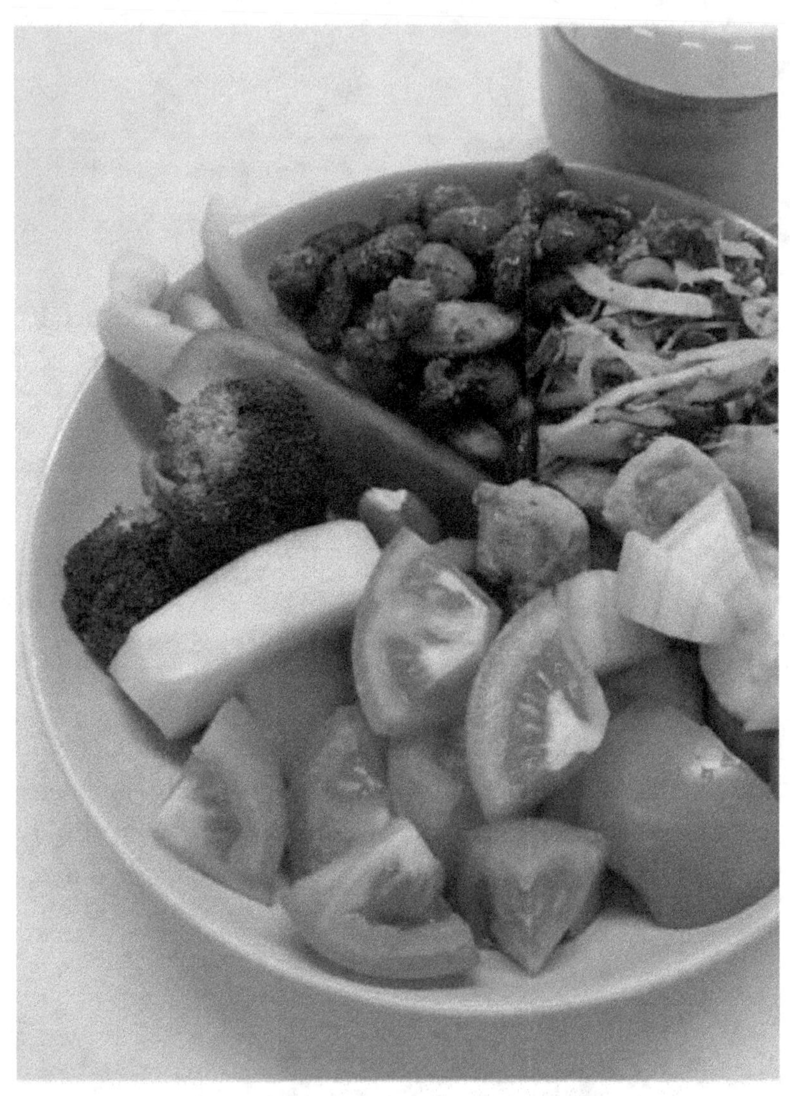

Chapter 6

10 Diabetic Renal Dinner Recipes

Here are ten diabetic renal dinner recipes along with their ingredients and preparation methods:

1. Baked Salmon with Lemon and Dill:

Ingredients:

- 1 salmon fillet
- Lemon slices
- Fresh dill
- Salt and pepper to taste

Preparation:

1. Preheat the oven to 375°F (190°C) and prepare a baking sheet with parchment paper.

2. Place the salmon fillet on the prepared baking sheet.

3. Season with salt and pepper.

4. Top with lemon slices and fresh dill.

5. Bake for 12-15 minutes, or until the salmon is done.

6. Serve hot.

2. Grilled Chicken Breast with Herbs:

Ingredients:

- Skinless, boneless chicken breast

- Mixed herbs (such as rosemary, thyme, and oregano)

- Salt and pepper to taste

Preparation:

1. Preheat the grill or grill pan on medium-high heat.

2. Season the chicken breast with mixed herbs, salt, and pepper.

3. Grill for 6-8 minutes on each side or until the chicken is cooked through.

4. Allow it to cool for a few minutes before slicing.

5. Serve hot.

3. Turkey and Vegetable Stir-Fry:

Ingredients:

- Lean ground turkey

- Assorted vegetables (such as bell peppers, broccoli, and snap peas)

- Low-sodium soy sauce

- Garlic powder

- Ginger powder

- Olive oil

Preparation:

1. Heat olive oil in a skillet or wok over medium-high heat.

2. Add the ground turkey and cook until browned.

3. Add the vegetables to the skillet and stir-fry until tender-crisp.

4. Season with garlic powder and ginger powder.

5. Stir in low-sodium soy sauce.

6. Cook for a few more minutes.

7. Serve immediately over brown rice or quinoa.

4. Baked Cod with Herbs and Lemon:

Ingredients:

- Cod fillets

- Mixed herbs (such as parsley, dill, and thyme)

- Lemon juice

- Salt and pepper to taste

Preparation:

1. Preheat the oven to 375 degrees Fahrenheit (190 degrees Celsius) and line a baking sheet with parchment paper.

2. Arrange the cod fillets on the prepared baking sheet.

3. Season with mixed herbs, lemon juice, salt, and pepper.

4. Bake for 12-15 minutes, or until the fish is well cooked and flakes readily with a fork.

5. Serve hot.

5. Grilled Shrimp Skewers:

Ingredients:

- Shrimp, peeled and deveined

- Lemon juice

- Garlic powder

- Paprika

- Olive oil

- Salt and pepper to taste

Preparation:

1. Preheat the grill or grill pan on medium-high heat.

2. In a bowl, combine the shrimp, lemon juice, garlic powder, paprika, olive oil, salt, and pepper.

3. Thread the shrimp onto skewers.

4. Grill for 2-3 minutes on each side or until the shrimp is pink and opaque.

5. Serve hot with a squeeze of lemon juice.

6. Baked Chicken Breast with Italian Seasoning:

Ingredients:

- Skinless, boneless chicken breast

- Italian seasoning

- Garlic powder

- Onion powder

- Salt and pepper to taste

Preparation:

1. Preheat the oven to 375°F (190°C) and line a baking sheet with parchment paper.

2. Place the chicken breast on the prepared baking sheet.

3. Season with Italian seasoning, garlic powder, onion powder, salt, and pepper.

4. Bake for 20-25 minutes, or until the chicken is thoroughly done.

5. Let it rest for a few minutes before serving.

6. Serve hot.

7. Baked Pork Tenderloin with Rosemary:

Ingredients:

- Pork tenderloin

- Fresh rosemary

- Garlic cloves, minced

- Olive oil

- Salt and pepper to taste

Preparation:

1. Preheat the oven to 375 degrees Fahrenheit (190 degrees Celsius) and line a baking sheet with parchment paper.

2. Rub the pork tenderloin with minced garlic, olive oil, salt, and pepper.

3. Sprinkle fresh rosemary over the pork.

4. Place the tenderloin on the prepared baking sheet.

5. Bake for 25-30 minutes or until the pork is cooked through and reaches an internal temperature of 145°F (63°C).

6. Allow it to cool for a few minutes before slicing.

7. Serve hot.

8. **Quinoa Pilaf with Mixed Vegetables:**

Ingredients:

- Cooked quinoa

- Vegetable mixture (like carrots, peas, and corn)

- Onion, chopped

- Garlic cloves, minced

- Low-sodium vegetable broth

- Olive oil

- Salt and pepper to taste

Preparation:

1. Heat olive oil in a skillet over medium heat.

2. Sauté the chopped onion and minced garlic until translucent.

3. Cook the mixed vegetables until tender..

1. Stir in the cooked quinoa and low-sodium vegetable broth.

2. Season with salt and pepper.

3. Cook for a few more minutes until the flavors are well combined.

4. Serve hot.

9. Barley Salad with Roasted Vegetables:

Ingredients:

- Cooked barley

- Assorted roasted vegetables (such as bell peppers, zucchini, and eggplant)

- Cherry tomatoes, halved

- Fresh basil leaves, torn

- Lemon vinaigrette dressing

Preparation:

1. In a bowl, combine the cooked barley, roasted vegetables, cherry tomatoes, and torn basil leaves.

2. Drizzle with lemon vinaigrette dressing and toss to coat.

3. Adjust seasoning if needed.

4. Serve chilled or at room temperature.

10. Lentil Soup:

Ingredients:

- Green or brown lentils, rinsed

- Onion, chopped

- Carrots, diced

- Celery, diced

- Garlic cloves, minced

- Low-sodium vegetable broth

- Dried thyme

- Olive oil

- Salt and pepper to taste

Preparation:

1. Get olive oil heated in a large pot over medium heat.

2. Sauté the chopped onion, diced carrots, diced celery, and minced garlic until softened.

3. Add the rinsed lentils, low-sodium vegetable broth, dried thyme, salt, and pepper.

4. Bring to a boil, then reduce the heat and simmer for 25-30 minutes or until the lentils are tender.

5. Adjust seasoning if needed.

6. Serve hot.

Remember to adjust the portion sizes and specific ingredients according to your dietary needs and any recommendations from your healthcare provider. Enjoy these dinner recipes as part of a balanced diabetic renal diet.

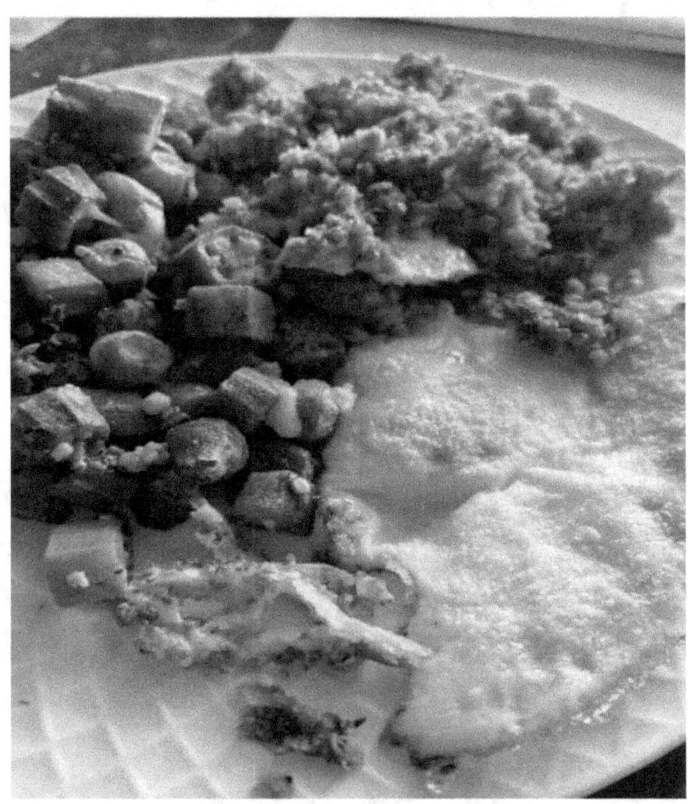

Conclusion

We hope that you have found inspiration, guidance, and satisfaction within its pages. This cookbook was created with the intention of supporting your health and well-being, providing you with a collection of flavorful recipes that meet the unique dietary needs of individuals with diabetes and renal conditions.

Throughout this journey, you have learned the importance of balancing your blood sugar levels and supporting your kidney function through mindful food choices. By incorporating the recipes from this cookbook into your daily routine, you have taken a proactive step towards managing your health in a delicious and nourishing way.

Remember that a diabetic renal diet is not just about restriction; it is about making informed choices and embracing a lifestyle that promotes wellness. We encourage you to continue exploring new flavors, ingredients, and cooking techniques. Adapt the recipes to suit your personal preferences and discover the joy of creating meals that both nourish your body and delight your taste buds.

It is crucial to remember that dietary changes are just one piece of the puzzle when it comes to managing your health. Consult with your healthcare provider, follow their recommendations, and integrate a comprehensive approach to your well-being, including exercise, medication management, and regular check-ups.

We would like to express our heartfelt gratitude for joining us on this culinary journey. We sincerely hope that this cookbook has provided you with the tools and inspiration to embrace a diabetic renal diet with confidence and joy. By nourishing your body, you are nurturing your overall health and embracing a lifestyle that promotes vitality and longevity.

As you continue your path towards a healthier you, we wish you strength, resilience, and the satisfaction of savoring each nourishing meal. Remember that every choice you make has the power to transform your health, and we believe in your ability to create a future filled with vitality and well-being.

Here's to nourishing meals and a life of vibrant health!

Bon appétit!